THE
ENDURING
TUBERCULOSIS

EXPLORING THE HISTORY OF OUR DEADLIEST DISEASE

JINNY VERMOS

To the millions who have suffered and succumbed to tuberculosis, and to the relentless researchers, doctors, and advocates who have worked tirelessly to combat its devastating grip. This book is a testament to your endurance and resilience.

Writing this book has been a journey into the depths of history, science, and humanity. I am profoundly grateful to the medical historians, archivists, and scientists who have devoted their lives to uncovering the truth about tuberculosis.

Special thanks to my editor, whose sharp insights shaped this book into what it is today, and to my family for their unwavering support during my research and writing. Finally, to the readers—may this book deepen your understanding of the world's most enduring epidemic and inspire action toward its eradication.

CONTENTS OF THIS BOOK

CHAPTER 1: A PLAGUE THROUGH THE AGES

Tuberculosis (TB) is not just a disease; it is a harrowing tale of survival, suffering, and resilience that spans millennia. As one of humanity's oldest recorded afflictions, TB has left an indelible mark on civilizations, shaping not only public health systems but also art, literature, and even cultural identities. Despite centuries of medical progress, the disease remains a formidable global health challenge, underscoring the intricate relationship between pathogens and human societies.

This chapter delves into the historical, social, and biological significance of tuberculosis, examining its persistence as a deadly global adversary.

The Silent Killer: Tuberculosis in Context

The unique danger of TB lies in its subtlety. Unlike the sudden outbreaks of plague or cholera, TB spreads quietly, often lying dormant for years before manifesting. Those infected may unknowingly pass the disease to others, creating a slow-moving epidemic that can persist for decades.

TB is caused by Mycobacterium tuberculosis, a bacterium that primarily attacks the lungs but can spread to the spine, brain, and other organs. The symptoms—chronic cough, fever, night sweats, and weight loss—paint a grim picture of its progression, but they often emerge too late, when the disease is already advanced.

What makes TB particularly dangerous is its ability to exploit vulnerabilities: poverty, malnutrition, and overcrowding provide the perfect breeding ground for its spread. It has thus become a disease of inequality, disproportionately affecting the marginalized and the poor.

Ancient Traces of Tuberculosis

Tuberculosis is as old as humanity itself. Archaeological evidence suggests that TB has been infecting humans for over 9,000 years. One of the earliest confirmed cases comes from a Neolithic burial site in the Eastern Mediterranean, where skeletons show telltale signs of spinal tuberculosis.

Mummies from ancient Egypt have provided further insights into TB's historical presence. The 3,300-year-old mummy of Pharaoh Akhenaten is believed to show skeletal evidence of TB, and ancient Egyptian texts describe symptoms consistent with the disease. In the Indian subcontinent, the ancient Ayurvedic texts, written around 1,500 BCE, describe a disease called "Rajayakshma" (king's disease), which bears remarkable similarities to TB.

Interestingly, TB's evolutionary history is tied closely to that of humans. Genetic studies suggest that Mycobacterium tuberculosis evolved from a bacterium that infected animals, possibly cattle, and adapted to humans as early as 70,000 years ago. This evolutionary relationship underscores the long-standing coexistence of TB with human societies.

A Disease Shrouded in Mystery

In ancient times, TB was poorly understood, often attributed to supernatural causes or divine punishment. Hippocrates, the "father of medicine," described TB as "phthisis," a wasting disease that was particularly common among young adults. He noted its contagious nature but believed it was caused by an imbalance in bodily humors, a theory that persisted for centuries.

In medieval Europe, TB was seen through a religious lens. The disease's wasting effects were interpreted as a sign of moral or spiritual failing. It was believed that saints could heal TB sufferers, and shrines dedicated to Saint Roch, the patron saint of plague and TB, became pilgrimage sites.

The Rise of the "White Death"

By the 17th and 18th centuries, TB had reached epidemic proportions in Europe. The Industrial Revolution, with its rapid urbanization and crowded living conditions, created the perfect storm for TB to thrive.

Cities like London and Paris saw staggering death rates, with TB accounting for one in four deaths during the 19th century.

The disease earned the nickname "White Death" due to the pale, ghostly appearance of its victims. It was also called "consumption," a reference to the way it seemed to consume the body from within, leaving patients emaciated and weakened.

Romanticizing Death: TB in Art and Literature

While TB was devastating, it paradoxically gained a romanticized reputation during the 19th century. Writers and artists saw the disease as a mark of creativity and sensitivity, associating it with heightened emotion and spiritual transcendence.

The poet John Keats, who succumbed to TB at the age of 25, became a symbol of this romantic ideal. His works, infused with themes of beauty and mortality, reflected his awareness of his impending death. Similarly, Emily Brontë, who wrote Wuthering Heights, and Frederic Chopin, the legendary composer, both died of TB, further cementing its association with genius.

However, this romanticization masked the true horror of TB. For every celebrated artist who died young, countless others suffered in silence, their lives cut short by the disease.

The Sanatorium Era

By the late 19th century, the medical community began to understand TB's contagious nature, leading to the establishment of sanatoriums.

These facilities, often located in rural areas, were designed to isolate TB patients and provide treatment through rest, fresh air, and nutrition.

Sanatoriums became a symbol of hope for some but were a source of stigma for others. For many patients, the isolation from family and society was a painful reminder of their exclusion. The sanatorium era also highlighted the class divide, as wealthier patients could afford private facilities, while the poor languished in overcrowded public institutions.

Koch's Breakthrough and the Antibiotic Era

In 1882, German scientist Robert Koch made a groundbreaking discovery: he identified Mycobacterium tuberculosis as the cause of TB. His work earned him a Nobel Prize and paved the way for modern treatments. However, it wasn't until the mid-20th century that effective antibiotics like streptomycin became widely available, dramatically reducing TB mortality rates.

Despite these advances, TB proved to be a resilient adversary. The emergence of drug-resistant strains in the late 20th century reignited fears of a global epidemic, reminding the world of TB's enduring threat.

Tuberculosis in the Modern World

Today, TB remains a global health crisis. The World Health Organization (WHO) estimates that one-quarter of the world's population is infected with latent TB, and over 10 million people develop active TB each year. The disease disproportionately affects low-income countries, where access to healthcare and treatment is limited.

The rise of multidrug-resistant TB (MDR-TB) and extensively drug-resistant TB (XDR-TB) has complicated efforts to control the disease. These strains, which do not respond to standard antibiotics, require expensive and toxic treatments that many patients cannot afford.

Furthermore, TB's close association with HIV/AIDS has created a deadly synergy. People with compromised immune systems are more susceptible to TB, and co-infection with HIV remains a leading cause of death in many regions, particularly sub-Saharan Africa.

A Disease That Reflects Humanity

TB is more than just a biological phenomenon; it is a mirror reflecting humanity's vulnerabilities, inequalities, and resilience. Its history reveals how social determinants—poverty, overcrowding, and stigma—have shaped its spread and treatment. At the same time, the fight against TB showcases humanity's capacity for innovation and cooperation.

This chapter is just the beginning of the journey into TB's complex history. The chapters that follow will explore its cultural, scientific, and medical dimensions, offering a comprehensive look at how this ancient disease continues to shape our world.

CHAPTER 2: EARLY TRACES: TUBERCULOSIS IN ANCIENT HISTORY

Tuberculosis (TB) has been a part of human history for so long that its origins predate written records. Long before modern medicine could identify its cause, TB silently stalked human populations, infecting and killing millions across generations. Evidence of its presence is etched into the bones of ancient humans and recorded in the earliest medical texts.

This chapter explores the ancient traces of TB, from archaeological discoveries to the disease's role in early societies. It highlights how humanity first encountered the "White Death" and how early civilizations understood and responded to this enduring adversary.

The Evolutionary Origins of Tuberculosis

TB is an ancient disease, not only in human history but also in evolutionary terms. Research suggests that Mycobacterium tuberculosis, the bacterium responsible for TB, evolved over 70,000 years ago, around the same time that modern humans were migrating out of Africa. Genetic studies indicate that TB likely originated as a zoonotic disease—one that jumped from animals to humans.

Early human populations living in close proximity to livestock may have contracted a form of TB from animals, such as cattle. This theory is supported by the genetic similarity between Mycobacterium tuberculosis and Mycobacterium bovis, which causes bovine TB. As humans migrated and formed larger, more settled communities, the disease adapted and spread among populations, becoming a persistent and deadly companion to humanity.

Archaeological Evidence: Tracing TB in Ancient Skeletons

One of the most compelling ways to study TB's ancient history is through skeletal remains. TB often leaves distinctive marks on the bones, particularly in cases of spinal tuberculosis (Pott's disease), where vertebrae collapse and fuse together.

Neolithic Burials: The First Traces of TB

The earliest confirmed evidence of TB comes from a 9,000-year-old skeleton discovered in the Eastern Mediterranean. This skeleton, belonging to a young adult, showed clear signs of spinal tuberculosis. Similar evidence has been found in other Neolithic burial sites, suggesting that TB was already present in early agricultural societies.

Egyptian Mummies: A Disease of the Pharaohs

Perhaps the most famous evidence of ancient TB comes from ancient Egypt. Mummies from the 18th and 19th dynasties (around 1,400 BCE) have been found with signs of tuberculosis, including spinal deformities and lung lesions. The mummified remains of Pharaoh Akhenaten and his family are particularly significant, as genetic testing has revealed traces of Mycobacterium tuberculosis.

Ancient Egyptian medical texts, such as the Ebers Papyrus, describe symptoms consistent with TB, including persistent cough and wasting. The Egyptians referred to the disease as "consumption" and attempted to treat it with herbal remedies and magical incantations, reflecting their belief in the spiritual origins of illness.

Pre-Columbian Americas: TB Before European Contact

Interestingly, TB was present in the Americas long before European colonization. Archaeologists have found evidence of TB in the remains of pre-Columbian peoples, including the Inca and Ancestral Puebloans. DNA analysis of ancient remains has confirmed that TB strains in the Americas were distinct from those in Europe, suggesting that the disease may have been transmitted through animal reservoirs or independent evolutionary pathways.

Tuberculosis in Ancient Medical Texts

While TB left physical marks on ancient bones, it also left an imprint in early medical literature. Across different cultures, TB was described in ways that reflected each society's understanding of health and disease.

India: Ayurveda and "Rajayakshma"

The ancient Indian medical system of Ayurveda contains some of the earliest written descriptions of TB. Known as "Rajayakshma" or "King's Disease," TB was characterized by wasting, coughing, and fever. Ayurvedic texts attributed the disease to an imbalance of the three doshas (vital energies) and prescribed a combination of herbal treatments, dietary changes, and spiritual practices to restore balance.

China: Ancient Remedies for "Lao Bing"

In ancient China, TB was referred to as "Lao Bing," meaning "wasting disease." Traditional Chinese Medicine (TCM) associated TB with an imbalance of yin and yang and the depletion of vital energy (qi). Treatments included acupuncture, herbal remedies, and dietary adjustments. The ancient Chinese also recognized the contagious nature of TB, advising patients to avoid close contact with others.

Greece and Rome: Hippocrates and Galen

In ancient Greece, the physician Hippocrates wrote extensively about TB, which he called "phthisis." He noted its prevalence among young adults and its characteristic symptoms, such as coughing, fever, and weight loss. However, like other ancient physicians, Hippocrates misunderstood the disease's cause, attributing it to an imbalance in bodily humors rather than an infectious agent.

The Roman physician Galen expanded on Hippocrates' work, describing TB as a disease of the lungs and offering treatments such as bloodletting and dietary modifications. Despite their limitations, these early medical texts laid the foundation for later understandings of TB.

Cultural and Spiritual Interpretations of TB

In ancient societies, TB was often viewed through a spiritual or supernatural lens. The wasting nature of the disease, combined with its mysterious and contagious qualities, made it a source of fear and fascination.

TB as a Curse or Punishment

Many ancient cultures believed that TB was a curse or punishment from the gods. This belief was particularly strong in societies where illness was seen as a reflection of moral or spiritual failings. In some cases, TB patients were ostracized or subjected to rituals aimed at purifying their souls.

The Healing Saints

In medieval Europe, TB patients often sought help from saints, particularly Saint Roch, the patron saint of plague and TB. Pilgrimages to shrines dedicated to Saint Roch were common, as people believed that his intercession could cure them of their afflictions.

The Impact of TB on Early Societies

The prevalence of TB in ancient societies had far-reaching effects on population dynamics, social structures, and cultural practices.

Urbanization and the Spread of TB

The rise of agriculture and the growth of cities created conditions that allowed TB to thrive. Overcrowded living spaces, poor sanitation, and close contact with livestock facilitated the spread of the disease. In many cases, TB became endemic, shaping the health and demographics of early urban populations.

TB and Social Inequality

Even in ancient times, TB disproportionately affected the poor and marginalized. Malnutrition and inadequate housing made certain populations more vulnerable to the disease, highlighting the links between TB and social inequality.

Lessons from the Past

The study of TB in ancient history reveals the enduring nature of the disease and humanity's long struggle to understand and combat it. While early societies lacked the scientific tools to identify the true cause of TB, their observations and attempts at treatment laid the groundwork for future discoveries.

As we move forward in this book, the ancient traces of TB provide a sobering reminder: this is not a new enemy, but one that has evolved alongside us for millennia. The persistence of TB in modern times is a testament to its adaptability and resilience—and a call to action for humanity to finally conquer this ancient foe.

CHAPTER 3: THE AGE OF DISCOVERY AND MISUNDERSTANDING

As humanity entered the Age of Discovery, tuberculosis (TB) persisted as one of the deadliest diseases across continents. From the late Middle Ages through the Renaissance and into the Enlightenment, this era was defined by progress in exploration, science, and medicine. Yet, TB, often referred to as "consumption" during this time, continued its silent conquest. Its victims included the wealthy and the poor, the powerful and the powerless, artists and laborers.

This chapter explores how societies from the 15th to 18th centuries grappled with TB. It examines the disease's entrenchment in social norms, its romanticization in art and literature, the early attempts at scientific understanding, and the tragic consequences of misguided treatments.

Tuberculosis in the Late Middle Ages

By the 15th century, tuberculosis was deeply entrenched in Europe. The crowded and unsanitary conditions of medieval towns created ideal conditions for its spread. The disease affected all social classes, although its impact on the poor was more severe due to malnutrition and lack of access to medical care.

Spiritual Interpretations: Sin and Salvation

In the deeply religious societies of the late Middle Ages, TB was often seen as a spiritual affliction. The disease's wasting effects—emaciated bodies, pale skin, and blood-tinged coughs—were interpreted as signs of divine punishment or moral failing. Many believed that TB was a consequence of sin, and its sufferers were sometimes ostracized or sent to isolated communities.

However, TB was also paradoxically associated with sanctity. Some saw the disease as a means of spiritual purification, likening its effects to the suffering of Christ. This duality—a disease of both sin and sanctity—shaped how societies treated those afflicted. Patients often turned to religious shrines, seeking miraculous cures through the intercession of saints such as Saint Roch or Saint Sebastian.

The Role of Urbanization

The late medieval period saw the growth of cities as centers of trade and commerce. Urbanization brought people into closer contact, accelerating the spread of TB. Crowded homes, shared wells, and poor ventilation created environments where the disease could thrive.

In many cities, TB became so common that it was almost an accepted part of life. It was referred to as "the wasting plague," and its presence was so pervasive that it often went unnoticed until it claimed the lives of loved ones.

The Renaissance: A Shift in Perception

The Renaissance ushered in an era of cultural and intellectual revival, but TB remained a constant presence. During this period, the disease began to influence art, literature, and even fashion, while early physicians sought to understand its causes.

The Romanticization of Consumption

The Renaissance saw a transformation in how TB was perceived, particularly among the upper classes. The disease's physical effects—pale skin, sunken cheeks, and slender figures—became associated with beauty and refinement. This romanticization of TB, especially among artists and poets, would later reach its peak in the 19th century.

TB in Art and Literature

The Renaissance fascination with death and mortality found a fitting metaphor in TB. The disease appeared in art and literature as a symbol of suffering, passion, and fragility. Paintings often depicted consumptive figures in states of quiet grace, their frailty evoking sympathy and admiration.

For example, in Shakespeare's plays, characters sometimes display symptoms of TB, reflecting its ubiquity in Elizabethan England. The Bard's intimate understanding of human frailty likely stemmed from observing TB's devastating effects on his contemporaries.

Early Medical Theories: The Four Humors

While the Renaissance celebrated human ingenuity, medical science was still in its infancy. TB was understood through the lens of the "four humors" theory, which posited that health depended on the balance of blood, phlegm, yellow bile, and black bile.

Physicians believed that TB was caused by an excess of phlegm, leading to treatments designed to restore balance. Bloodletting, purging, and dietary restrictions were common practices, but they often weakened patients further, hastening their deaths. Despite their limitations, Renaissance physicians laid the groundwork for later discoveries, emphasizing observation and experimentation.

The Enlightenment: Early Scientific Insights

The Enlightenment brought significant advances in science and medicine, yet TB continued to baffle researchers. The period saw the first attempts to classify diseases systematically, as well as new theories about the nature of infection and contagion.

The Rise of Contagion Theories

During the 17th and 18th centuries, some physicians began to suspect that TB was contagious. Observations of its spread within families and communities suggested that the disease could be transmitted from person to person. However, these theories were controversial and met with resistance from those who clung to older ideas about miasmas (bad air) as the cause of disease.

The Italian physician Girolamo Fracastoro was one of the first to propose a germ theory of disease in his 1546 work De Contagione et

Contagiosis Morbis. Although he did not specifically identify TB, his ideas laid the groundwork for future discoveries.

Misguided Treatments and Quackery

While some Enlightenment physicians made genuine progress in understanding TB, others promoted harmful or ineffective treatments. "Cures" ranged from inhaling the smoke of burned herbs to consuming mercury-based tonics. Wealthy patients were often prescribed trips to the countryside or seaside, where fresh air and rest were believed to restore health.

For the poor, treatments were often more brutal. Bloodletting and purging remained common, while some patients were subjected to "sweating therapies" in hot rooms designed to expel toxins. These interventions, based on flawed theories, often caused more harm than good.

Tuberculosis and the Age of Exploration

The Age of Exploration (15th to 17th centuries) played a significant role in the global spread of TB. European explorers, traders, and colonizers carried the disease to new territories, where it wreaked havoc on indigenous populations.

The Impact on Indigenous Peoples

In the Americas, Australia, and the Pacific Islands, TB devastated communities that had no prior exposure to the disease. Indigenous populations, lacking immunity to Mycobacterium tuberculosis, experienced mortality rates as high as 90% in some regions.

The introduction of TB by European colonizers compounded the effects of other diseases, such as smallpox and measles, contributing to the collapse of many indigenous societies. These tragic events underscore TB's role in the broader narrative of colonialism and exploitation.

The Cultural Legacy of Tuberculosis

By the end of the 18th century, TB had become deeply embedded in the cultural fabric of Europe and beyond. Its presence shaped not only medical practices but also societal attitudes toward illness, death, and beauty.

TB as a Social Equalizer

Although TB disproportionately affected the poor, it did not spare the wealthy. Kings, queens, artists, and intellectuals all fell victim to the disease, reinforcing the idea that TB was a universal threat. This perception helped foster a sense of shared vulnerability, even as it highlighted the inequalities that exacerbated the disease's spread.

The Seeds of Future Discoveries

The Enlightenment's emphasis on observation, experimentation, and skepticism laid the foundation for the scientific breakthroughs of the 19th century. While TB remained a mystery, the intellectual groundwork was being laid for its eventual understanding.

Conclusion: A Pervasive Mystery

The Age of Discovery and Misunderstanding was a period of progress and paradox. Humanity expanded its knowledge of the world, yet TB remained a formidable and poorly understood adversary. The disease's romanticization in art and literature contrasted sharply with its devastating reality, while early scientific efforts offered hope even as they fell short of providing solutions.

As we move into the 19th century in the next chapter, we will see how the Industrial Revolution and the rise of modern science transformed humanity's battle against tuberculosis. The foundations laid during this era would ultimately lead to the breakthroughs that changed the course of the disease—but not without further suffering and loss.

CHAPTER 4: THE INDUSTRIAL REVOLUTION: TUBERCULOSIS AND THE RISE OF MODERN MEDICINE

The Industrial Revolution marked one of the most transformative periods in human history. From the late 18th to the early 19th century, technological advancements reshaped societies, economies, and environments. However, this progress came at a cost. Urbanization, industrialization, and poor living conditions created a perfect storm for the spread of tuberculosis (TB). The disease thrived in overcrowded slums, factories, and poorly ventilated homes, leading to an unprecedented surge in its prevalence and mortality.

In this chapter, we delve into the devastating impact of TB during the Industrial Revolution, the early public health responses, and the birth of modern medicine. This period saw the disease evolve from being a misunderstood affliction to the focus of groundbreaking scientific discoveries, paving the way for future interventions.

The Perfect Storm: Tuberculosis in the Age of Urbanization

The Industrial Revolution was synonymous with rapid urban growth. Millions of people migrated from rural areas to cities in search of work, resulting in densely populated urban centers. These cities, often unprepared for such an influx, became breeding grounds for diseases like TB.

Overcrowded Slums and Squalor

In cities like London, Manchester, Paris, and New York, the living conditions of the working class were deplorable. Families were crammed into single-room tenements, often without proper ventilation or sanitation. Damp, dark, and unhygienic environments facilitated the spread of TB. The disease was so rampant that it earned the nickname "the White Plague," a reference to the pale, wasted appearance of its victims.

The rise of factory work further exacerbated the problem. Factory laborers, including women and children, worked long hours in poorly ventilated and dust-filled environments. The cramped conditions in factories not only exposed workers to TB but also weakened their immune systems, making them more susceptible to the disease.

The Unequal Burden of Disease

Although TB affected all social classes, its impact was disproportionately severe on the poor. Malnutrition, overwork, and lack of access to medical care created a vicious cycle of poverty and illness. Wealthier individuals, while not immune, had the means to escape urban centers and seek treatment in the countryside or abroad.

This stark inequality underscored the social determinants of health and the role of systemic factors in the spread of disease.

Early Public Health Responses

The explosion of TB cases during the Industrial Revolution spurred some of the first organized public health efforts. Governments, physicians, and reformers began to recognize the need for collective action to combat the disease.

Sanitation and Hygiene Movements

One of the earliest responses to the TB epidemic was the sanitation movement. Reformers like Edwin Chadwick in England and Rudolph Virchow in Germany advocated for improved living conditions, clean water, and proper waste disposal. Their work led to the establishment of public health boards and the construction of sewer systems, which, while not directly targeting TB, helped reduce overall disease burden.

The Advent of Hospital Care

During this period, hospitals began to play a more significant role in the treatment of TB patients. Sanatoriums, specialized institutions for TB care, also emerged as a response to the growing epidemic. These facilities emphasized rest, fresh air, and a nutritious diet, based on the belief that such measures could help patients recover. The sanatorium movement gained traction in Europe and North America, offering hope to thousands of patients, though its efficacy was limited.

Contagion vs. Miasma Theories

Debates about the nature of TB shaped early public health policies. While some physicians argued that TB was contagious, others adhered to the miasma theory, which attributed the disease to "bad air" from decaying organic matter. This lack of consensus hindered efforts to control the disease. It was not until the late 19th century that the germ theory of disease, championed by scientists like Louis Pasteur and Robert Koch, provided definitive evidence of TB's infectious nature.

TB and the Rise of Modern Medicine

The Industrial Revolution coincided with significant advancements in medical science, many of which were driven by the need to understand and combat TB.

The Work of René Laennec

One of the most important figures in the history of TB during this period was René Laennec, a French physician who invented the stethoscope in 1816. Laennec used his invention to study lung diseases, including TB, and documented his findings in his seminal work De l'Auscultation Médiate. His detailed descriptions of TB's pathological effects on the lungs advanced medical knowledge and improved diagnostic techniques.

Pathological Studies and Autopsies

The practice of performing autopsies became more widespread during the Industrial Revolution, providing valuable insights into the physical manifestations of TB. Physicians observed the characteristic tubercles (small, rounded nodules) in the lungs and other organs of deceased patients, confirming that TB was a systemic disease.

Early Attempts at Vaccination

While a vaccine for TB would not be developed until the 20th century, the success of Edward Jenner's smallpox vaccine in 1796 inspired early experiments in immunization. Some physicians speculated that exposure to cowpox or other animal diseases might confer immunity to TB, though these theories remained unproven at the time.

Tuberculosis in Literature and Art

The cultural impact of TB during the Industrial Revolution cannot be overstated. The disease was a recurring theme in literature, art, and music, reflecting its pervasive presence in society.

Romanticizing the White Plague

In the 19th century, TB became closely associated with the Romantic movement. The disease was often depicted as a "poetic" affliction, its victims portrayed as sensitive, artistic souls whose suffering elevated them to a higher plane of existence. This romanticization was fueled by the fact that many prominent artists and writers, including John Keats, Percy Bysshe Shelley, and Frédéric Chopin, succumbed to TB.

TB in Victorian Literature

Victorian novels frequently featured characters suffering from TB, using the disease as a metaphor for moral or emotional turmoil. Charles Dickens, for example, depicted TB in Nicholas Nickleby through the character of Smike, whose physical decline mirrors his tragic circumstances. Similarly, Elizabeth Gaskell's Ruth explores the social stigma and emotional impact of the disease.

Artistic Representations

Paintings from the Industrial Revolution era often depicted the effects of TB, from emaciated bodies to pale, ethereal faces. These artworks served as both a reflection of societal fears and a testament to the resilience of those who endured the disease.

The Industrial Revolution's Global Impact on TB

While the Industrial Revolution began in Europe, its effects were felt worldwide. The spread of industrialization and colonialism carried TB to new regions, where it took a devastating toll on indigenous populations.

TB in Colonized Lands

European colonizers brought TB to Africa, Asia, and the Americas, where it ravaged communities with no prior exposure to the disease. In many cases, TB became a leading cause of death, exacerbating the social and economic disruption caused by colonial exploitation.

Urbanization in Developing Nations

As industrialization spread to developing nations, the same patterns of urbanization, overcrowding, and poverty that fueled TB in Europe were replicated elsewhere. By the late 19th century, TB had become a global epidemic, affecting every corner of the world.

The Legacy of the Industrial Revolution

The Industrial Revolution's impact on TB was profound and multifaceted. It exacerbated the disease's spread through urbanization and poor living conditions, but it also laid the groundwork for modern medicine and public health. The period's scientific discoveries, cultural reflections, and early interventions set the stage for the breakthroughs of the 20th century.

Conclusion: A Turning Point

The Industrial Revolution was a turning point in the history of TB. It highlighted the complex interplay between social, economic, and environmental factors in the spread of disease, while also spurring advances in science and medicine. As we move into the next chapter, we will explore the golden age of microbiology and the revolutionary discoveries that transformed our understanding of TB—and brought us closer to conquering it.

CHAPTER 5: THE GOLDEN AGE OF MICROBIOLOGY: UNVEILING TUBERCULOSIS

The late 19th and early 20th centuries marked a pivotal moment in the history of tuberculosis (TB). Known as the "Golden Age of Microbiology," this period was characterized by groundbreaking discoveries in medical science that unraveled the mysteries of many infectious diseases, including TB. For centuries, humanity had battled this silent killer without understanding its true nature. However, with advancements in microbiology, the tide began to turn.

This chapter delves into the remarkable discoveries that emerged during this era, focusing on the identification of the causative agent of TB, the development of diagnostic techniques, and the scientific revolution that forever changed medicine's approach to infectious diseases. The contributions of scientists like Robert Koch, Louis Pasteur, and others are explored in detail, as are the societal and medical impacts of their work.

Tuberculosis Before Koch's Breakthrough

Before the late 19th century, TB was a poorly understood disease. Although it was widely recognized as a leading cause of death, its origins and transmission remained shrouded in mystery. Many still clung to outdated theories, such as the miasma theory, which attributed the disease to "bad air."

Competing Theories of Disease

By the mid-19th century, the scientific community was divided over the nature of infectious diseases. While some believed that diseases were caused by microorganisms, others argued for alternative explanations, including hereditary predisposition or environmental factors. TB, in particular, was often thought to result from a combination of poor living conditions and weak constitutions.

Early Observations of Contagion

Despite the lack of scientific evidence, there were observations suggesting that TB might be contagious. Physicians noted its tendency to spread within families and close communities. However, without a clear understanding of the mechanisms of transmission, these observations were often dismissed or misunderstood.

Robert Koch and the Discovery of Mycobacterium Tuberculosis

The turning point in the fight against TB came in 1882 when German physician and microbiologist Robert Koch identified the bacterium responsible for the disease. His discovery was a monumental achievement that earned him the Nobel Prize in Physiology or Medicine in 1905.

The Road to Discovery

Koch's journey to uncover the cause of TB began with his pioneering work on anthrax. Building on the germ theory of disease proposed by Louis Pasteur, Koch developed innovative techniques for isolating and studying microorganisms. His meticulous methods included staining bacteria with dyes to make them visible under a microscope, a breakthrough that would prove crucial in identifying Mycobacterium tuberculosis.

Using his staining techniques, Koch demonstrated the presence of the TB bacillus in tissue samples from infected patients. He then fulfilled the postulates that now bear his name—Koch's Postulates—by isolating the bacterium, cultivating it in a lab, and showing that it caused TB when introduced into experimental animals.

The Impact of Koch's Discovery

Koch's identification of Mycobacterium tuberculosis revolutionized medicine. For the first time, TB was understood as an infectious disease caused by a specific microorganism, not a vague result of poor living conditions or moral failing. This discovery paved the way for targeted diagnostic techniques, treatments, and public health measures.

The Rise of Diagnostic Techniques

With the identification of Mycobacterium tuberculosis, the focus shifted to diagnosing the disease accurately and efficiently. Early diagnostic methods laid the foundation for modern approaches still in use today.

Sputum Microscopy

One of the first diagnostic tools developed after Koch's discovery was sputum microscopy. By examining the sputum of suspected TB patients under a microscope, physicians could identify the characteristic TB bacilli. This method, though labor-intensive, provided a reliable way to confirm a diagnosis.

The Tuberculin Skin Test

In 1890, Koch introduced tuberculin, a protein extract derived from Mycobacterium tuberculosis. Although initially intended as a treatment, tuberculin proved ineffective for curing TB. However, it later became the basis for the tuberculin skin test, a diagnostic tool that detects an individual's immune response to TB infection. This test remains widely used today, particularly in screening programs.

Louis Pasteur and the Germ Theory Revolution

While Robert Koch is often credited with the discovery of the TB bacillus, his work was part of a broader scientific movement spearheaded by Louis Pasteur. Pasteur's germ theory of disease provided the conceptual framework for understanding infectious diseases, including TB.

Pasteur's Contributions

Pasteur's experiments in the 1860s demonstrated that microorganisms were responsible for fermentation and spoilage. He extended these findings to medicine, arguing that specific germs caused specific diseases. This groundbreaking insight laid the foundation for the field of microbiology and inspired a generation of scientists to study pathogens like Mycobacterium tuberculosis.

Vaccination as a Concept

Although Pasteur did not develop a vaccine for TB, his work on vaccines for other diseases, such as rabies and anthrax, influenced future efforts to create immunizations against TB. The concept of vaccination gained widespread acceptance during this period, setting the stage for the eventual development of the Bacillus Calmette-Guérin (BCG) vaccine in the 20th century.

Public Health Responses and Sanitation

The discoveries of Koch, Pasteur, and their contemporaries had a profound impact on public health policies. Governments and medical institutions began to implement measures aimed at controlling the spread of TB.

Isolation and Sanatoriums

Recognizing the contagious nature of TB, public health officials advocated for the isolation of infected individuals. Sanatoriums, which had been gaining popularity during the Industrial Revolution, became central to TB control efforts. These institutions provided patients with fresh air, rest, and nutritious food, reflecting the belief that a healthy environment could aid recovery.

While sanatoriums did little to cure TB, they helped slow its spread by isolating infectious patients. They also played a role in raising awareness about the disease and fostering early research into its treatment.

Public Education Campaigns

Public health campaigns began to emphasize the importance of hygiene and disease prevention. Posters and pamphlets urged citizens to cover their mouths when coughing, avoid spitting in public, and seek medical attention for persistent coughs. These campaigns, though rudimentary by modern standards, marked an important step toward disease control.

The Societal Impact of Scientific Discoveries

The Golden Age of Microbiology not only transformed medicine but also had far-reaching effects on society. TB, once shrouded in mystery and superstition, became the subject of rigorous scientific inquiry.

Shifting Perceptions of Disease

The identification of Mycobacterium tuberculosis helped dispel many of the myths surrounding TB. It was no longer seen as a hereditary curse or a moral failing but as an infectious disease that could potentially be controlled and treated. This shift in perception reduced some of the stigma associated with TB, though discrimination against patients persisted in many communities.

A Catalyst for Research

Koch's work inspired a wave of research into other infectious diseases, leading to the identification of pathogens responsible for cholera, typhoid, and diphtheria, among others. The scientific breakthroughs of this era laid the foundation for modern microbiology, immunology, and epidemiology.

The Limitations of Early Discoveries

Despite the progress made during the Golden Age of Microbiology, many challenges remained. Effective treatments for TB were still decades away, and the disease continued to claim millions of lives. The lack of antibiotics and vaccines meant that prevention and isolation remained the primary strategies for controlling TB.

Conclusion: A Scientific Revolution

The Golden Age of Microbiology was a transformative period in the fight against TB. The discovery of Mycobacterium tuberculosis by Robert Koch, combined with the broader contributions of Louis Pasteur and others, marked the beginning of a new era in medicine. For the first time, humanity had the tools to understand TB at a fundamental level, setting the stage for future breakthroughs in treatment and prevention.

As we move into the 20th century in the next chapter, we will explore how these scientific advances were translated into practical solutions. From the development of antibiotics to the creation of vaccines, the 20th century would bring humanity closer than ever to defeating tuberculosis.

Chapter 6: The 20th Century: War, Medicine, and the Fight Against Tuberculosis

As the world entered the 20th century, tuberculosis (TB) remained one of humanity's deadliest diseases. Despite the scientific breakthroughs of the late 19th century, including Robert Koch's identification of

Mycobacterium tuberculosis, TB continued to ravage populations across the globe. The disease's persistence was a stark reminder that understanding its cause was only the first step in combating it.

This chapter explores the key developments in TB control during the early to mid-20th century, from the creation of the Bacillus Calmette-Guérin (BCG) vaccine to the discovery of life-saving antibiotics like streptomycin. It also examines the social, political, and economic forces that shaped global efforts to combat TB, including the role of two World Wars and the establishment of international health organizations.

The World Wars and Their Impact on Tuberculosis

The early decades of the 20th century were marked by unprecedented global conflict, with World War I (1914–1918) and World War II (1939–

1945) reshaping societies, economies, and public health systems. These wars had a profound impact on the fight against TB.

Tuberculosis in the Trenches

During World War I, TB became a significant health concern for soldiers and civilians alike. The cramped, unsanitary conditions of trenches provided an ideal environment for the disease to spread. Soldiers weakened by malnutrition, fatigue, and stress were particularly vulnerable. Military hospitals struggled to care for TB patients, and many soldiers were discharged from service due to the disease's debilitating effects.

On the home front, wartime hardships exacerbated TB's impact. Food shortages, overcrowded housing, and limited access to medical care increased the disease's prevalence among civilian populations. Women and children, often left behind while men went to war, were disproportionately affected.

World War II and Advances in Medicine

World War II brought both challenges and opportunities in the fight against TB. On one hand, the war disrupted public health systems and diverted resources away from disease control efforts. On the other hand, it spurred significant advancements in medical science. The need to care for wounded soldiers and prevent infectious diseases led to increased investment in research and the development of new treatments, including antibiotics.

The BCG Vaccine: A Preventive Breakthrough

One of the most significant milestones in the fight against TB was the development of the Bacillus Calmette-Guérin (BCG) vaccine.

The Origins of BCG

The BCG vaccine was developed by French scientists Albert Calmette and Camille Guérin in the early 1920s. Using a weakened strain of Mycobacterium bovis (a close relative of Mycobacterium tuberculosis), they created a vaccine that stimulated the immune system to fight TB without causing the disease.

The first human trial of the BCG vaccine took place in 1921, and its use gradually expanded over the following decades. By the mid-20th century, the BCG vaccine had become a cornerstone of global TB prevention efforts, particularly in countries with high disease burdens.

Successes and Limitations

While the BCG vaccine proved effective in preventing severe forms of TB, such as meningitis in children, its efficacy in preventing pulmonary TB—the most common and infectious form—was variable. Factors such as geographic location, genetic diversity, and prior exposure to other mycobacteria influenced the vaccine's effectiveness. Despite these limitations, the BCG vaccine remains widely used and has saved millions of lives.

The Discovery of Antibiotics: A Turning Point

The mid-20th century witnessed the development of antibiotics that revolutionized the treatment of TB.

Streptomycin: The First TB Antibiotic

In 1943, American microbiologist Selman Waksman and his colleagues discovered streptomycin, the first effective antibiotic for TB. Streptomycin directly targeted Mycobacterium tuberculosis, killing the bacteria and dramatically improving patient outcomes. Its introduction in 1944 marked a turning point in TB treatment, transforming a once-fatal disease into a manageable condition for many patients.

Combination Therapy and Drug Resistance

Although streptomycin was a breakthrough, it soon became apparent that TB bacteria could develop resistance to the drug when used alone. This led to the development of combination therapy, which involved using multiple antibiotics simultaneously to prevent resistance. By the 1950s, other antibiotics, such as isoniazid and pyrazinamide, had been introduced, forming the basis of modern TB treatment regimens.

Global Public Health Campaigns

The mid-20th century saw the emergence of large-scale public health campaigns aimed at controlling TB. These efforts were driven by international organizations, national governments, and local health authorities.

The Role of the World Health Organization

Founded in 1948, the World Health Organization (WHO) quickly identified TB as a major global health priority. The WHO launched a series of initiatives to improve TB diagnosis, treatment, and prevention. These included mass vaccination campaigns with the BCG vaccine, as well as the establishment of TB treatment programs in low- and middle-income countries.

Mass Screening and Radiography

Advances in medical technology enabled mass screening programs for TB. Mobile X-ray units were deployed to identify cases in communities, factories, and schools. Early detection allowed for timely treatment, reducing transmission and mortality.

Community-Based Approaches

In addition to medical interventions, public health campaigns emphasized education and community involvement. Posters, pamphlets, and radio broadcasts informed the public about TB symptoms, prevention, and treatment. Community health workers played a key role in identifying cases and supporting patients through their treatment journeys.

Challenges and Inequities

Despite significant progress, the fight against TB during the 20th century was fraught with challenges.

Inequities in Access to Care

Access to TB diagnosis and treatment varied widely between and within countries. While wealthier nations benefited from advanced medical technologies and well-funded health systems, many low-income countries struggled to provide basic care. Rural and marginalized communities often faced barriers to accessing treatment, perpetuating cycles of disease and poverty.

Stigma and Discrimination

The stigma surrounding TB remained a significant obstacle to control efforts. Many patients faced discrimination in their communities and workplaces, deterring them from seeking care. Public health campaigns sought to combat stigma by promoting understanding and empathy, but progress was slow.

The End of the Era

By the 1960s, TB mortality rates had declined dramatically in many parts of the world, thanks to antibiotics, vaccination, and improved living conditions. However, the disease was far from eradicated. TB persisted in regions with high poverty, overcrowding, and weak health systems. Moreover, the emergence of drug-resistant strains posed a new and formidable challenge.

Conclusion: A Fragile Victory

The early to mid-20th century was a period of remarkable progress in the fight against TB. The development of the BCG vaccine, the discovery of antibiotics, and the implementation of global public health campaigns saved countless lives and transformed the landscape of TB control. However, these victories were fragile, as the disease continued to exploit social and economic vulnerabilities.

As we move into the latter half of the 20th century and beyond, the story of TB becomes one of both hope and caution. The next chapter will explore the rise of drug-resistant TB, the impact of the HIV/AIDS epidemic, and the ongoing efforts to achieve a world free of tuberculosis. .

CHAPTER 7: THE RISE OF DRUG-RESISTANT TUBERCULOSIS

The mid-20th century brought unprecedented advances in the fight against tuberculosis (TB). With antibiotics like streptomycin, isoniazid, and rifampicin becoming widely available, it seemed as though the world might finally overcome one of humanity's deadliest diseases. However, by the late 20th century, a new threat emerged that would challenge this progress: drug-resistant tuberculosis (DR-TB).

This chapter explores the origins, spread, and impact of drug-resistant TB, as well as the global response to this growing crisis. It examines the scientific, social, and economic factors that contributed to the rise of DR-TB and highlights the ongoing struggle to develop new treatments and strategies to combat it.

Understanding Drug-Resistant Tuberculosis

Drug-resistant TB occurs when Mycobacterium tuberculosis develops the ability to survive treatment with one or more antibiotics. This resistance can occur naturally through genetic mutations or as a result of improper or incomplete treatment.

Types of Drug Resistance

- Monoresistant TB: Resistance to a single first-line drug, such as isoniazid or rifampicin.

- Multidrug-Resistant TB (MDR-TB): Resistance to at least isoniazid and rifampicin, the two most powerful first-line antibiotics.

- Extensively Drug-Resistant TB (XDR-TB): Resistance to isoniazid, rifampicin, fluoroquinolones, and at least one second-line injectable drug, such as amikacin or kanamycin.

- Totally Drug-Resistant TB (TDR-TB): Rare cases where the bacteria are resistant to all available TB drugs.

The Origins of Drug Resistance

Drug-resistant TB was first identified in the 1940s, shortly after the introduction of streptomycin. However, it wasn't until the 1980s and 1990s that it became a major public health crisis.

The Role of Mismanagement

Improper use of antibiotics played a significant role in the development of drug resistance. Factors included:

- Incomplete Treatment: Patients stopping their medication prematurely due to side effects, financial constraints, or feeling better.

- Incorrect Prescriptions: Healthcare providers prescribing the wrong drugs, doses, or treatment durations.

- Unregulated Antibiotic Use: Over-the-counter access to TB drugs in many countries allowed patients to self-medicate without proper guidance.

The Global Spread of Resistance

The rapid globalization of the late 20th century facilitated the spread of drug-resistant TB. Increased international travel and migration, particularly from high-burden areas, allowed resistant strains to cross borders. In many cases, conflict, poverty, and weak healthcare systems exacerbated the problem.

The HIV/AIDS Epidemic and Its Impact

The HIV/AIDS epidemic of the 1980s and 1990s created a perfect storm for the resurgence of TB, including drug-resistant forms.

A Deadly Combination

HIV weakens the immune system, making individuals more susceptible to TB infection and progression from latent TB to active disease. Co-infection with TB and HIV became a leading cause of death among people living with HIV/AIDS, particularly in sub-Saharan Africa.

Amplifying Drug Resistance

The high burden of TB in HIV-positive populations placed immense pressure on healthcare systems. Overcrowded clinics and limited resources often led to inconsistent treatment, fueling the emergence of drug-resistant strains.

The Social and Economic Costs

Drug-resistant TB imposes a heavy burden on individuals, families, and societies.

The Cost of Treatment

Treating drug-resistant TB is significantly more expensive and complex than treating drug-susceptible TB. MDR-TB treatment requires a combination of second-line drugs, which are less effective, more toxic, and must be taken for longer periods—often 18 to 24 months. These treatments can cost thousands of dollars per patient, far beyond the reach of many in low-income settings.

The Human Toll

Patients with drug-resistant TB often endure severe side effects, including hearing loss, nausea, and mental health challenges. The prolonged treatment regimen disrupts their lives, preventing them from working or caring for their families. Stigma and discrimination further isolate patients, compounding their suffering.

Economic Impact

At the societal level, drug-resistant TB strains healthcare systems, reduces workforce productivity, and hampers economic development. In high-burden countries, the economic losses associated with TB can reach billions of dollars annually.

Scientific and Medical Responses

The rise of drug-resistant TB prompted an urgent global response, with researchers, policymakers, and healthcare providers working to develop new tools and strategies.

New Diagnostic Tools

Advances in molecular biology led to the development of rapid diagnostic tests, such as the Xpert MTB/RIF assay. Introduced in 2010, this test detects TB and rifampicin resistance in under two hours, allowing for quicker diagnosis and treatment.

New Treatment Regimens

In recent years, shorter and more effective regimens for drug-resistant TB have been developed. For example:

- Bedaquiline: Approved in 2012, this drug targets ATP synthase, a critical enzyme in TB bacteria.

- Delamanid: Another new drug that inhibits cell wall synthesis in Mycobacterium tuberculosis.

- The BPaL Regimen: A combination of bedaquiline, pretomanid, and linezolid that offers a shorter treatment duration for XDR-TB.

Research into Vaccines

Efforts to develop more effective TB vaccines are ongoing. While the BCG vaccine remains in use, its limited efficacy against pulmonary TB has spurred the search for new candidates. Several promising vaccine candidates are currently in clinical trials.

Global Public Health Initiatives

The fight against drug-resistant TB has become a priority for international organizations, governments, and NGOs.

The WHO's End TB Strategy

Launched in 2014, the WHO's End TB Strategy aims to reduce TB deaths by 95% and new cases by 90% by 2035. The strategy emphasizes:

- Early diagnosis and treatment of drug-resistant TB.

- Strengthening healthcare systems in high-burden countries.

- Investing in research and innovation.

The Green Light Committee

Established by the WHO in 2000, the Green Light Committee helps countries access affordable, quality-assured second-line drugs for MDR-TB. By improving treatment access, the committee aims to curb the spread of resistance.

Community-Based Approaches

Engaging communities in TB control efforts has proven essential. Community health workers play a critical role in supporting patients through their treatment, reducing stigma, and promoting prevention.

Challenges and the Road Ahead

Despite significant progress, the fight against drug-resistant TB is far from over.

Barriers to Access

Many patients in low- and middle-income countries still lack access to diagnostics, treatment, and supportive care. Addressing these disparities is crucial to achieving global TB control.

The Threat of Totally Drug-Resistant TB

The emergence of TDR-TB highlights the urgent need for new antibiotics and treatment strategies. Without these tools, the world risks losing the progress made over the past century.

Sustained Political Will

Ending drug-resistant TB requires sustained political and financial commitment at both national and international levels. Advocacy efforts must continue to prioritize TB as a global health emergency.

Conclusion: A Battle Yet to Be Won

The rise of drug-resistant TB is a stark reminder that the fight against tuberculosis is not over. While scientific and medical advancements have provided powerful tools, their success depends on equitable access, robust healthcare systems, and global collaboration.

As we move forward, the lessons learned from the past must guide our efforts. Only through sustained commitment and innovation can we hope to overcome the challenge of drug-resistant TB and move closer to a world free of this enduring disease.

Chapter 8: Tuberculosis and the HIV/AIDS Syndemic

The late 20th century saw tuberculosis (TB) become intertwined with another devastating global health crisis: the HIV/AIDS epidemic. The syndemic—where two diseases interact to worsen their collective impact—created a deadly partnership that claimed millions of lives, particularly in sub-Saharan Africa. TB, already a persistent public health challenge, experienced a resurgence in regions with high HIV prevalence.

This chapter explores the relationship between TB and HIV/AIDS, examining how the two diseases amplify each other's effects, the public health challenges they present, and the global response to this dual epidemic. It also highlights the human stories behind the statistics, shedding light on the struggles faced by individuals, communities, and healthcare systems.

The Intersection of TB and HIV/AIDS

The term "syndemic" aptly describes the relationship between TB and HIV. Unlike a mere co-infection, a syndemic involves diseases that interact to exacerbate each other's impact. For people living with HIV,

TB became the leading cause of death, with the two diseases forming a vicious cycle.

How HIV Increases TB Risk

HIV weakens the immune system by attacking CD4 T-cells, which play a critical role in defending the body against infections. This immunosuppression makes individuals more vulnerable to latent TB infection progressing to active disease. In fact, people living with HIV are 18 times more likely to develop active TB than those without HIV.

How TB Worsens HIV Outcomes

TB not only accelerates HIV progression but also complicates its treatment. The inflammation caused by active TB increases viral replication, leading to higher HIV viral loads. Additionally, drug interactions between TB treatments and antiretroviral therapy (ART) pose significant challenges for healthcare providers and patients.

The Global Burden of TB/HIV Co-Infection

Sub-Saharan Africa: The Epicenter

Sub-Saharan Africa became the epicenter of the TB/HIV syndemic in the late 20th and early 21st centuries. The region's high HIV prevalence, combined with socio-economic factors like poverty, overcrowding, and weak healthcare systems, created ideal conditions for the resurgence of TB. Countries like South Africa, Zimbabwe, and Eswatini reported some of the highest rates of TB/HIV co-infection globally.

Other High-Burden Regions

While sub-Saharan Africa bore the brunt of the syndemic, other regions, including Southeast Asia and Eastern Europe, also faced significant challenges. In Eastern Europe, the rise of multidrug-resistant TB (MDR-TB) compounded the impact of HIV, creating a particularly dire public health crisis.

Challenges in Managing the TB/HIV Syndemic

Diagnostic Difficulties

Diagnosing TB in people living with HIV is often more complex than in HIV-negative individuals. HIV-positive patients frequently present with atypical TB symptoms, and the disease may be more difficult to detect on chest X-rays. Moreover, the traditional sputum smear microscopy test has reduced sensitivity in immunocompromised patients.

The development of rapid diagnostic tools, such as the GeneXpert MTB/RIF assay, has improved detection, but these technologies remain inaccessible in many resource-limited settings.

Treatment Complications

Managing TB and HIV simultaneously requires careful coordination of treatment regimens. Key challenges include:

- Drug Interactions: Rifampicin, a cornerstone of TB treatment, reduces the efficacy of certain antiretroviral drugs, necessitating dose adjustments or alternative therapies.

- Adherence Issues: Patients with TB/HIV co-infection face complex treatment regimens, often involving dozens of pills per day. This increases the risk of non-adherence, leading to drug resistance and treatment failure.

- Immune Reconstitution Inflammatory Syndrome (IRIS): Starting ART in patients with advanced HIV and active TB can trigger IRIS, a potentially life-threatening inflammatory response as the immune system begins to recover.

Stigma and Discrimination

Stigma surrounding both TB and HIV poses significant barriers to diagnosis, treatment, and prevention. Many patients face social isolation, discrimination, and loss of employment, deterring them from seeking care. This stigma is particularly pronounced in communities where TB and HIV are associated with poverty and "moral failings."

The Global Response to the TB/HIV Syndemic

Recognizing the devastating impact of the TB/HIV syndemic, the global health community mobilized to address the dual epidemic.

Collaborative Frameworks

In 2004, the World Health Organization (WHO) and UNAIDS launched the "Interim Policy on Collaborative TB/HIV Activities," which outlined strategies for integrating TB and HIV services. These included:

- Offering HIV testing and counseling to all TB patients.

- Screening all HIV-positive individuals for TB.

- Providing preventive therapy for latent TB infection in people living with HIV.

- Ensuring coordinated treatment for patients with TB/HIV co-infection.

Antiretroviral Therapy and TB Prevention

The widespread rollout of ART in the early 2000s transformed HIV care and had a significant impact on TB prevention. By suppressing HIV viral loads and restoring immune function, ART reduces the risk of TB reactivation in people living with HIV.

Additionally, the use of isoniazid preventive therapy (IPT) has been shown to significantly reduce the risk of active TB in HIV-positive individuals with latent infection.

Funding and Advocacy

International funding mechanisms, such as the Global Fund to Fight AIDS, Tuberculosis, and Malaria, played a crucial role in scaling up TB and HIV services. These initiatives provided financial and technical support to high-burden countries, enabling them to expand access to diagnostics, treatment, and prevention.

Non-governmental organizations (NGOs) and community-based organizations also played a vital role in advocating for patient rights, reducing stigma, and delivering care to marginalized populations.

Success Stories and Lessons Learned

Progress in Sub-Saharan Africa

Several countries in sub-Saharan Africa achieved significant progress in reducing TB/HIV co-infection rates. For example:

- South Africa: Through aggressive scale-up of ART and IPT, South Africa halved its TB incidence rate between 2008 and 2018.

- Eswatini: Once the country with the highest TB/HIV co-infection rate, Eswatini implemented integrated TB/HIV services and achieved dramatic improvements in patient outcomes.

Lessons for Future Epidemics

The TB/HIV response provided valuable lessons for managing future health crises:

- The importance of integrating services for co-existing diseases.

- The need for sustained political and financial commitment.

- The value of community engagement and patient-centered care.

Ongoing Challenges

Despite progress, the TB/HIV syndemic remains a significant global health challenge.

Persistent Inequities

Access to TB and HIV services remains uneven, with rural and marginalized communities often left behind. Closing these gaps is essential to achieving equitable health outcomes.

Drug-Resistant TB

The rise of MDR-TB and extensively drug-resistant TB (XDR-TB) poses a major threat to the fight against TB/HIV co-infection. Addressing this challenge requires continued investment in research, diagnostics, and treatment.

Stigma and Social Determinants

Tackling the social determinants of health, such as poverty, housing, and education, is critical to addressing the root causes of the TB/HIV syndemic.

Conclusion: A Dual Epidemic, A Shared Solution

The TB/HIV syndemic has been one of the most complex and devastating health crises of the late 20th and early 21st centuries. However, it has also demonstrated the power of global collaboration, scientific innovation, and community-driven solutions.

As the world continues to battle TB and HIV, the lessons learned from this dual epidemic will serve as a blueprint for addressing future public health challenges. By investing in integrated care, reducing stigma, and addressing social inequities, we can move closer to a future free from the devastating impact of TB and HIV.

CHAPTER 9: THE EVOLUTION OF TUBERCULOSIS IN THE MODERN WORLD

Tuberculosis (TB), a disease that has plagued humanity for centuries, continues to shape the global health landscape even in the 21st century. While significant strides have been made in its control and treatment, the disease's persistence, adaptability, and the emergence of new challenges keep it a major public health threat. This chapter explores the evolution of tuberculosis in the modern world, focusing on the factors that have allowed the disease to endure, the contemporary scientific and medical approaches to combating it, and the ongoing struggles that hinder global TB control.

The State of Tuberculosis in the 21st Century

Despite the dramatic decrease in TB mortality rates in many parts of the world, the disease remains a leading cause of death worldwide. According to the World Health Organization (WHO), TB continues to be the second leading infectious killer globally, after COVID-19, with over 10 million people falling ill with TB every year. Over 1.5 million people die from the disease annually, the vast majority of whom live in low- and middle-income countries.

The Persistent Threat of Tuberculosis

While high-income countries have seen substantial declines in TB incidence, low- and middle-income countries, particularly in sub-Saharan Africa, Southeast Asia, and Eastern Europe, remain the epicenter of the global TB burden. In these regions, TB thrives in contexts of overcrowded living conditions, inadequate healthcare infrastructure, poor nutrition, and weak public health systems. These socio-economic factors, combined with the persistent problem of TB-related stigma, continue to hinder TB control efforts.

The Challenge of Emerging Strains

Modern-day TB is not simply a continuation of the disease we have known for centuries; it has evolved in response to changing environmental conditions and the widespread use (and misuse) of antibiotics. The emergence of drug-resistant strains of Mycobacterium tuberculosis, such as multidrug-resistant TB (MDR-TB) and extensively drug-resistant TB (XDR-TB), has added a new layer of complexity to efforts to control the disease.

The Impact of Globalization and Urbanization

The forces of globalization and urbanization have played a significant role in the spread and persistence of TB. As the world becomes more interconnected, people travel more frequently across borders, carrying with them not only their ideas and cultures but also the potential for spreading infectious diseases like TB.

Migration and Mobility

Global migration, both voluntary and forced, has contributed to the spread of TB in regions where it may have previously been under control. Refugees and migrants from countries with high TB burdens often live in crowded, resource-poor conditions, which increases the risk of TB transmission. These populations may also face barriers to accessing healthcare and proper TB treatment, further compounding the problem.

In high-income countries, migrants from TB-endemic regions are disproportionately affected by the disease, highlighting the global nature of the epidemic. This situation demands international cooperation and coordination in TB prevention, diagnosis, and treatment efforts.

The Urbanization Factor

As more people around the world migrate to urban areas in search of work and better living conditions, urbanization has become a significant factor in TB transmission. Overcrowded slums and informal settlements, often lacking adequate sanitation and healthcare infrastructure, provide a fertile breeding ground for TB bacteria. In these environments, the disease spreads easily among people who are already vulnerable due to poor nutrition, underlying health conditions, or compromised immune systems.

Advances in TB Diagnosis and Treatment

Despite the persistent challenges, the field of TB diagnosis and treatment has seen significant advancements in the modern world. The development of new diagnostic tools, more effective treatments, and a growing understanding of TB's molecular biology has brought hope to the fight against the disease.

Rapid Diagnostic Technologies

One of the most important advancements in modern TB control has been the development of rapid diagnostic tests. Traditional methods of diagnosing TB, such as sputum smear microscopy and chest X-rays, can be time-consuming, require specialized equipment, and often miss cases of drug-resistant TB. New molecular diagnostic technologies, such as the GeneXpert MTB/RIF assay, allow for faster and more accurate diagnosis of TB and rifampicin resistance, enabling healthcare providers to start appropriate treatment sooner.

GeneXpert, for example, can provide results within two hours, significantly reducing the diagnostic delay that has traditionally been associated with TB testing. This has been particularly valuable in high-burden, resource-poor settings where timely diagnosis is critical to preventing further transmission.

Shorter and More Effective Treatment Regimens

For many years, TB treatment consisted of a lengthy regimen of first-line drugs, often taken for six months or longer. However, recent advances in TB treatment have focused on shortening treatment durations while maintaining high efficacy. For drug-resistant TB, second-line drugs are used, but these treatments can be complex, require longer durations, and are often accompanied by serious side effects.

New drug regimens are changing this landscape. For example, the introduction of shorter regimens for MDR-TB has been a significant breakthrough. The BPaL regimen, which combines bedaquiline, pretomanid, and linezolid, offers a shorter treatment course, with promising results in clinical trials. Bedaquiline, in particular, has been a game-changer in the fight against drug-resistant TB. It targets an enzyme essential for TB bacteria to generate energy, preventing the bacteria from reproducing and spreading.

Vaccination Efforts

The development of a more effective TB vaccine remains one of the most pressing priorities in TB research. While the BCG vaccine has been in use since the 1920s and provides some protection against severe forms of TB in children, it is only partially effective in preventing pulmonary TB in adults, the most common and contagious form of the disease.

In recent years, several vaccine candidates have entered clinical trials, including M72/AS01E, a candidate that showed promising results in preventing TB infection in people at high risk, such as those living with HIV. These new vaccine developments offer hope for reducing the global TB burden, particularly in areas where TB transmission is rampant.

The Role of Drug-Resistant TB in the Modern World

While advancements in TB treatment are promising, the rise of drug-resistant TB remains one of the most significant threats to global TB control. Multidrug-resistant TB (MDR-TB) and extensively drug-resistant

TB (XDR-TB) are difficult to treat and require expensive, toxic second-line drugs.

MDR-TB: A Growing Crisis

MDR-TB is defined as resistance to at least isoniazid and rifampicin, the two most powerful first-line antibiotics used to treat TB. The emergence of MDR-TB has been fueled by the improper use of antibiotics, incomplete treatment regimens, and the lack of access to quality healthcare in many parts of the world. MDR-TB not only complicates treatment but also increases the risk of transmission, as individuals with untreated MDR-TB are highly infectious.

XDR-TB: A Dire Situation

XDR-TB is a more severe form of resistance, characterized by resistance to both first-line and second-line antibiotics, including fluoroquinolones and injectable drugs like amikacin. Treatment for XDR-TB is extremely limited, with only a few effective drugs available. XDR-TB has a high mortality rate, and managing it often requires long, costly treatment courses, with limited success in many cases.

As global TB incidence begins to decline, the threat of drug-resistant TB looms larger. MDR-TB and XDR-TB pose a challenge not only in terms of treatment complexity but also in terms of surveillance, as these strains may go undetected until they are widespread.

The Economic and Social Burden of Tuberculosis

Tuberculosis, particularly drug-resistant forms, places a heavy economic burden on individuals, families, and societies. The cost of diagnosis, treatment, and the loss of productivity due to illness can be devastating, especially in low-income regions.

Economic Costs of TB Treatment

The financial cost of treating TB, especially drug-resistant forms, is substantial. For MDR-TB, treatment regimens can cost thousands of dollars per patient, far beyond the means of many individuals in resource-limited settings. This not only impacts the patient but also places a significant strain on national healthcare budgets. In countries with high TB burdens, the economic toll of TB can undermine efforts to address other health issues, as resources are diverted to TB control programs.

Social Impact and Stigma

Beyond the financial costs, TB carries a significant social burden. The stigma associated with TB, particularly drug-resistant forms, can lead to social isolation, discrimination, and mental health challenges for affected individuals. In many cultures, TB is seen as a shameful disease, and patients may be ostracized or blamed for their condition. This stigma can discourage people from seeking treatment, leading to further transmission and exacerbating the problem.

Moving Forward: The Path to Ending Tuberculosis

While the road ahead remains challenging, there are signs of hope in the global effort to end TB. International initiatives, such as the WHO's "End TB Strategy," aim to reduce TB deaths by 95% and new cases by 90% by 2035.

Strengthening Health Systems

To achieve these ambitious targets, countries must strengthen their healthcare systems. This includes improving TB surveillance, ensuring access to diagnostic tools and treatments, and building the capacity of health workers to diagnose and manage TB effectively.

Global Collaboration

Ending TB will require continued global cooperation. High-income countries must support TB control efforts in low- and middle-income countries through financial aid, technology transfer, and capacity-building initiatives. The private sector, research institutions, and non-governmental organizations all have roles to play in advancing TB research and treatment options.

Tackling Social Determinants

The fight against TB cannot be won by healthcare systems alone. Addressing the social determinants of health, such as poverty,

Housing, nutrition, and education, is essential to reducing TB transmission and ensuring equitable access to treatment.

Conclusion: A Shared Global Responsibility

The modern world's battle with tuberculosis is far from over. While advancements in medicine, diagnostics, and treatment have led to significant improvements, the rise of drug-resistant strains, combined with the social and economic factors that perpetuate the disease, ensures that TB remains a formidable opponent.

The global response to tuberculosis must continue to evolve, integrating scientific innovation with community-based solutions. By confronting TB's root causes—poverty, inadequate healthcare, stigma, and social inequities—and investing in the tools and resources necessary for effective diagnosis and treatment, we can move closer to a world free of TB.

In the fight against tuberculosis, no one is exempt. It is a global responsibility, one that requires international solidarity, political will, and a commitment to health equity. Only by working together can we hope to bring an end to one of humanity's oldest and deadliest diseases.

CHAPTER 10: THE SEARCH FOR A CURE – SCIENTIFIC BREAKTHROUGHS IN THE FIGHT AGAINST TUBERCULOSIS

The quest to find a cure for tuberculosis (TB) has been a long and arduous journey, marked by scientific breakthroughs, failed experiments, and relentless pursuit by researchers, doctors, and healthcare workers. Although TB has been a constant presence in human history, the scientific community has made significant strides in understanding the disease and developing treatments. Despite these advances, TB remains a global health threat, and the search for an effective cure continues. This chapter delves into the scientific breakthroughs that have shaped the fight against TB, the challenges that remain, and the ongoing efforts to eradicate the disease once and for all.

Early Attempts and the Discovery of the Causative Agent

The story of TB's treatment begins in the 19th century, when the disease was still largely misunderstood. Early attempts to cure TB were based on rudimentary ideas, ranging from herbal remedies to invasive surgeries. TB was often regarded as an incurable disease, and patients who developed symptoms were often left to suffer without effective medical intervention.

The Rise of Germ Theory

The first significant scientific breakthrough in the fight against TB came in 1882 when the German physician Robert Koch discovered the bacterium Mycobacterium tuberculosis, the causative agent of TB. Koch's identification of the bacterium revolutionized our understanding of the disease, shifting it from a vague concept of "consumption" to a clear-cut infectious disease. His discovery earned him the Nobel Prize in Physiology or Medicine in 1905, but it also raised more questions about how to effectively treat and cure the disease.

Koch's work was foundational in the development of diagnostic methods such as the tuberculin skin test, which helped detect latent TB infections. However, at the time, there were still no effective treatments, and TB remained a major public health crisis.

The Discovery of the First TB Drugs

After Koch's discovery, researchers began to focus on finding treatments to combat M. tuberculosis. The first breakthrough came in the 1940s with the discovery of streptomycin, an antibiotic that proved effective in treating TB. This discovery marked a turning point in the fight against TB, as it was the first drug to significantly reduce mortality from the disease. Streptomycin was introduced as a treatment for TB in 1944, and its success led to the development of additional antibiotics, including para-aminosalicylic acid (PAS) and isoniazid, which became the backbone of TB therapy for several decades.

However, despite the success of these drugs, TB remained a significant public health issue due to the long duration of treatment and the emergence of drug resistance. As more people were treated, it became apparent that improper use of antibiotics, such as incomplete courses of treatment, was leading to the development of drug-resistant strains of M. tuberculosis.

The Rise of Multidrug-Resistant TB (MDR-TB)

The emergence of multidrug-resistant TB (MDR-TB) in the 1980s and 1990s posed a major setback in the fight against TB. MDR-TB refers to strains of M. tuberculosis that are resistant to at least the two most powerful first-line drugs, isoniazid and rifampicin. The rise of MDR-TB was largely attributed to the misuse and overuse of antibiotics, particularly in settings where TB diagnosis and treatment were inadequate. In some cases, patients failed to complete their treatment regimens, leading to the development of resistant strains that were far more difficult to treat.

MDR-TB presented new challenges for the global TB response, as the existing drugs and treatment protocols were no longer effective. The search for new drugs and therapies became a top priority in the fight against TB.

The Discovery of New Drugs and Treatment Regimens

In response to the growing threat of drug-resistant TB, the scientific community intensified its efforts to develop new drugs and treatment regimens. Over the last two decades, several new drugs have been introduced to combat TB, particularly drug-resistant forms of the disease. These include bedaquiline, delamanid, and pretomanid, which represent significant advancements in the treatment of MDR-TB and extensively drug-resistant TB (XDR-TB).

Bedaquiline: A Game-Changer in TB Treatment

Bedaquiline, approved in 2012, is one of the most promising new drugs for treating drug-resistant TB. It works by inhibiting the ATP synthase enzyme, which is essential for the bacteria's energy production, effectively halting its growth and replication. Bedaquiline is especially effective against MDR-TB and XDR-TB strains, providing hope for patients who would otherwise face limited treatment options.

While bedaquiline has shown significant efficacy in clinical trials, its use is still limited by concerns about side effects, such as liver toxicity and the potential for heart arrhythmias. As a result, it is typically used in combination with other drugs and under close medical supervision.

Delamanid and Pretomanid

Delamanid and pretomanid are two other new drugs approved for the treatment of MDR-TB. Both drugs work by targeting the cell wall of M. tuberculosis, disrupting its ability to grow and divide. Pretomanid, in particular, has shown efficacy in a combination regimen with bedaquiline and linezolid, offering a shorter treatment course for MDR-TB patients.

These newer drugs have raised hopes for shortening treatment durations and improving outcomes for MDR-TB patients. However, their high cost and limited availability in low-resource settings remain significant barriers to widespread use.

The Role of the TB Vaccine: BCG and Beyond

The development of a more effective vaccine remains one of the most critical areas of TB research. While the Bacillus Calmette-Guérin (BCG) vaccine has been in use since the 1920s, it has limited efficacy in preventing pulmonary TB in adults—the most contagious and deadly form of the disease. As a result, the search for a more effective vaccine has remained a key priority for researchers.

The BCG Vaccine

The BCG vaccine is still widely used, particularly in countries with a high burden of TB, to prevent severe forms of TB in children, such as TB meningitis and miliary TB. However, its effectiveness in preventing adult pulmonary TB is variable, with some studies showing protection rates as low as 50%. Because of these limitations, researchers have focused on developing new vaccines that offer better protection against the most common and contagious form of TB.

New Vaccine Candidates

Several new TB vaccine candidates are currently in development, and some are showing promising results in clinical trials. One such candidate, M72/AS01E, has demonstrated an ability to prevent TB infection in individuals with a high risk of developing active disease, such as those living with HIV. In addition, researchers are exploring vaccines that combine multiple components of M. tuberculosis, targeting various stages of the bacteria's life cycle.

While these new vaccines show promise, their widespread use is still years away, as they require more extensive testing and regulatory approval. Nonetheless, the potential for a more effective vaccine represents a crucial part of the future of TB prevention.

The Role of Diagnostic Advancements in TB Control

Advances in TB diagnostics have been another key area of scientific progress. Early TB detection is critical to preventing transmission and ensuring that patients receive the appropriate treatment. However, traditional diagnostic methods, such as sputum smear microscopy, are often inaccurate, particularly in detecting drug-resistant strains of TB.

Molecular Diagnostics

Recent advancements in molecular diagnostics have revolutionized TB testing. The GeneXpert MTB/RIF test, introduced in 2010, provides a rapid and accurate way to diagnose TB and detect rifampicin resistance in a matter of hours. This has been a game-changer, particularly in low-resource settings, where traditional diagnostic methods were slow and unreliable.

In addition to GeneXpert, new molecular tools are being developed to detect TB more quickly and accurately. These include next-generation sequencing technologies that can identify drug-resistant mutations with high sensitivity. These diagnostic tools allow healthcare providers to tailor treatment regimens more effectively and reduce the risk of transmission by identifying infectious individuals earlier.

The Challenges of TB Drug Development

Despite these advancements, the development of new TB drugs and vaccines faces significant challenges. Drug development is an expensive and time-consuming process, and pharmaceutical companies often lack the financial incentive to invest in TB research, given the relatively low profit potential in developing countries with high TB burdens.

The Role of Public-Private Partnerships

To address this gap, public-private partnerships have played a critical role in funding and accelerating TB drug development. Organizations such as the Global Fund to Fight AIDS, Tuberculosis, and Malaria, along with the Bill & Melinda Gates Foundation and the Stop TB Partnership, have provided substantial financial support for TB research and development. These collaborations are essential for ensuring that the most promising new drugs and vaccines reach the market, especially for patients with drug-resistant TB who are in desperate need of new treatment options.

The Need for Comprehensive Approaches

Although scientific breakthroughs are crucial in the fight against TB, a comprehensive approach is needed to end the disease. This includes not only improving diagnosis, treatment, and prevention but also addressing the underlying social determinants of health, such as poverty, overcrowding, and lack of access to healthcare. TB control must be integrated into broader health systems, with an emphasis on equity and access for all populations.

Conclusion: Hope for the Future of TB Treatment and Cure

The journey toward a cure for tuberculosis is far from over, but the progress made over the past century offers hope for the future. From the discovery of the TB bacterium to the development of new drugs and vaccines, science has made tremendous strides in understanding and combating the disease. However, challenges remain, particularly with the rise of drug-resistant TB and the need for

More effective vaccines.

The fight against tuberculosis requires continued innovation, collaboration, and investment. The global response must go beyond medical treatments, addressing the social and economic factors that perpetuate the spread of TB. With ongoing scientific breakthroughs and a commitment to global health equity, the dream of a world free from tuberculosis is within reach.

Chapter 11: Addressing the Social Determinants – The Intersection of Poverty, Stigma, and Tuberculosis

The battle against tuberculosis (TB) is not solely one of medical advancements and scientific discoveries. Equally significant in reducing its impact is addressing the underlying social determinants that fuel the spread of the disease. Poverty, inadequate housing, malnutrition, and limited access to healthcare exacerbate the conditions under which TB thrives. Meanwhile, stigma—both surrounding the disease itself and its sufferers—compounds the difficulties of controlling TB, preventing people from seeking care and adhering to treatment. This chapter explores how social factors influence the TB epidemic, examining how poverty, social inequality, and stigma intersect to perpetuate the spread of the disease. It also considers strategies for tackling these social challenges in tandem with medical interventions.

The Social Context of Tuberculosis: A Global Perspective

Tuberculosis has always been a disease closely linked to social conditions, particularly poverty. For centuries, TB has disproportionately affected vulnerable populations, those living in crowded, unsanitary conditions with inadequate access to nutrition and healthcare. Today, despite advances in medical science, TB continues to ravage communities in areas with high levels of poverty and social inequality.

In high-burden TB countries, the prevalence of the disease is often highest in marginalized groups: those living in informal settlements, slums, or rural areas with limited infrastructure. Migrants, prisoners, people living with HIV, and those suffering from malnutrition are also more susceptible to TB due to the intersection of social, environmental, and biological factors. The global nature of TB is evident in the way the disease disproportionately affects low- and middle-income countries, where the resources to effectively diagnose, treat, and prevent TB are often limited.

Addressing the root causes of TB requires an understanding of the structural inequalities and social factors that contribute to its transmission. The role of poverty in perpetuating TB is multifaceted, influencing everything from the living conditions of individuals to their ability to access healthcare.

Poverty and Tuberculosis: A Vicious Cycle

Poverty is one of the primary drivers of the global TB epidemic. People living in poverty are more likely to be exposed to the bacteria that causes TB due to overcrowded housing, poor ventilation, and limited access to healthcare services. Poverty also increases susceptibility to TB by compromising the immune system. Malnutrition, common in impoverished communities, weakens the body's ability to fight infections, making it easier for Mycobacterium tuberculosis to take hold.

Overcrowded and Poor Housing Conditions

Many TB hotspots are located in densely populated urban slums or rural areas where people live in close quarters with limited space, poor ventilation, and substandard sanitation. These conditions create the ideal environment for TB transmission, as the bacteria spreads through the air when an infected person coughs or sneezes. Without adequate housing or the resources to improve living conditions, individuals are continually exposed to the risks of TB.

Access to Healthcare and Diagnostics

Poverty is also a barrier to accessing timely and effective TB diagnosis and treatment. In low-income areas, healthcare systems are often under-resourced and overburdened, making it difficult for individuals to access necessary medical services. Many people in poverty may not have the financial means to seek care, or they may live too far from healthcare facilities to access them regularly. In such contexts, TB cases often go undiagnosed, leading to delayed treatment and further spread of the disease within communities.

For those living in rural or remote areas, reaching diagnostic centers can be especially challenging. In many parts of the world, there is a shortage of trained healthcare workers and diagnostic equipment, which compounds the difficulty of identifying and treating TB cases early.

The Intersection of HIV and Tuberculosis: Amplifying the Crisis

The coexistence of HIV and TB is another critical issue in the fight against tuberculosis. HIV weakens the immune system, making individuals more susceptible to contracting TB. It is estimated that people living with HIV are up to 30 times more likely to develop active TB than those without HIV. The HIV epidemic, which began in the 1980s, has contributed to the rise of TB in regions with high HIV prevalence.

In some countries, particularly in sub-Saharan Africa, the overlap of the two diseases has led to a situation where TB is one of the leading causes of death among people living with HIV. The co-infection of TB and HIV presents additional challenges for treatment, as both diseases require different types of care, medication, and management strategies. In many resource-poor settings, the lack of integration between TB and HIV services can lead to poor outcomes for individuals with both conditions.

Moreover, antiretroviral therapy (ART), while critical for managing HIV, can sometimes complicate TB treatment. Many TB drugs interact with ART, leading to increased side effects and potential treatment failure if not managed carefully. This complex interaction underscores the need for integrated treatment approaches that address both TB and HIV simultaneously, particularly in high-burden settings.

Stigma and Tuberculosis: Barriers to Care

In addition to the structural and biological factors that contribute to TB's spread, stigma plays a significant role in delaying diagnosis and treatment. TB has long been associated with social stigma, partly due to its infectious nature and the misconceptions surrounding its transmission. Historically, TB was often seen as a disease of the poor, the homeless, and those with weakened immune systems. In many cultures, people with TB are viewed with fear or judgment, leading them to hide their symptoms and avoid seeking medical attention.

Fear of Isolation and Discrimination

The social stigma surrounding TB can be severe, particularly in communities where the disease is associated with poverty or marginalization. Individuals diagnosed with TB may face discrimination in their communities, workplaces, or even within their families. Fear of being ostracized can discourage people from seeking diagnosis and treatment, thereby increasing the risk of transmitting the disease to others.

This stigma is particularly acute in areas where TB is intertwined with HIV. People who are co-infected with both TB and HIV often experience compounded stigma. In many societies, HIV/AIDS is associated with behaviors considered morally unacceptable, such as drug use or sex work, and those living with HIV often face discrimination as well. For individuals diagnosed with both TB and HIV, the double burden of stigma can be overwhelming, leading them to avoid healthcare settings altogether.

The Impact of Stigma on Treatment Adherence

Stigma also significantly impacts treatment adherence. People with TB may feel embarrassed or ashamed to disclose their diagnosis, leading to inconsistent treatment regimens. TB treatment often requires taking multiple medications for an extended period, sometimes for months or even years, which can be challenging in the face of stigma. Those who fear discrimination may stop taking their medications, or they may not seek treatment at all, prolonging their illness and increasing the risk of drug resistance.

Healthcare workers must be trained to approach TB patients with sensitivity and compassion, creating a supportive environment where patients feel comfortable disclosing their diagnosis and adhering to treatment. Community-based programs that educate the public about TB and combat misconceptions can also play a crucial role in reducing stigma and encouraging people to seek care.

The Role of Education and Advocacy in Addressing Social Determinants

Tackling the social determinants of TB requires a multifaceted approach, combining public health interventions, education, and advocacy. Education plays a pivotal role in raising awareness about TB, its transmission, and its prevention. By reducing the stigma associated with the disease and providing accurate information, public health campaigns can encourage people to seek diagnosis and treatment early.

Community-Led Interventions

Community-based programs have proven to be effective in addressing the social determinants of TB. In many high-burden countries, local organizations and activists have played a crucial role in educating the public, providing support to TB patients, and advocating for better healthcare services. These programs often focus on vulnerable groups, including women, children, migrants, and people living with HIV, ensuring that they have access to the care they need.

For example, community health workers are often the first point of contact for individuals with TB in rural or underserved areas. These workers provide education about TB prevention, assist with diagnostic referrals, and help patients navigate the healthcare system. By engaging communities directly, these programs help break down the barriers to care caused by poverty and stigma.

Addressing the Social and Economic Conditions

Beyond healthcare interventions, addressing the social and economic conditions that drive TB is essential. Poverty reduction strategies, such as improving access to housing, clean water, and nutrition, are crucial in preventing TB transmission. Social protection programs that provide financial support to vulnerable populations can also help alleviate the economic burden of the disease, allowing individuals to seek care and follow through with treatment.

Conclusion: A Comprehensive Approach to Ending TB

The fight against tuberculosis requires a comprehensive approach that goes beyond medical treatment and diagnosis. By addressing the social determinants of health—such as poverty, inadequate housing, and malnutrition—alongside tackling stigma and discrimination, we can create a more effective response to the TB epidemic.

Public health efforts must prioritize social equity, ensuring that vulnerable populations have access to the resources and care they need to combat TB. This requires collaboration across sectors, including healthcare, education, housing, and social welfare, as well as strong political will to address the root causes of the disease.

Ultimately, ending the TB epidemic is not just a matter of advancing medical science, but also of creating a more just and equitable world, where everyone has the opportunity to live free from the burden of disease.

CHAPTER 12: THE FUTURE OF TUBERCULOSIS: INNOVATIONS, CHALLENGES, AND GLOBAL COMMITMENT

As the world continues to grapple with the persistence of tuberculosis (TB), the future of its control and eradication hinges on a multifaceted approach that includes scientific innovation, social reform, and global collaboration. Despite being one of the oldest known diseases, TB remains a significant public health challenge. However, the ongoing advancements in research, technology, and treatment offer hope that the end of the TB epidemic may one day be achievable. This chapter explores the innovations on the horizon for TB diagnosis, treatment, and prevention, as well as the ongoing challenges that must be overcome. It also highlights the importance of global commitment and action in the fight against TB, emphasizing the need for sustained investment and international cooperation.

Innovations in Tuberculosis Diagnosis: From Old to New Technologies

One of the key barriers to effectively controlling tuberculosis is the delay in diagnosing the disease, particularly in resource-limited settings. Traditional diagnostic methods, while still in use, can be slow, inaccurate, and costly. Over the years, however, there has been significant progress in the development of more efficient, rapid, and accessible diagnostic tools. These innovations hold the potential to transform the way TB is detected and treated worldwide.

Molecular Diagnostics: A Leap Forward in Speed and Accuracy

Molecular diagnostics have revolutionized the ability to detect TB quickly and accurately. Tests like the GeneXpert, which detects the presence of TB bacteria and identifies drug-resistant strains within hours, have made it possible for healthcare providers to begin treatment almost immediately. GeneXpert is now widely used in countries with high TB burdens, reducing the diagnostic delay that was once a major obstacle in controlling the disease. These molecular tools are particularly valuable in detecting drug-resistant TB, a growing threat in the global fight against TB.

Other molecular technologies, such as CRISPR-based diagnostics and next-generation sequencing, hold promise for even more rapid and accurate detection. These tools offer the potential to identify TB bacteria at the genetic level, providing detailed information on the specific strain of TB and its resistance profile. Such detailed insights can guide more personalized treatment plans and contribute to more effective management of the disease.

Artificial Intelligence and Digital Health

The integration of artificial intelligence (AI) and digital health technologies is opening new avenues for TB diagnosis and monitoring.

AI-powered algorithms are being developed to analyze chest X-rays and CT scans, identifying signs of TB even in the earliest stages of infection. These systems can assist radiologists in interpreting medical images more efficiently, reducing the time required for diagnosis.

Digital health platforms are also being utilized for remote monitoring of TB patients. Through mobile apps and telemedicine, healthcare providers can track patient adherence to treatment regimens, offer guidance, and intervene if there are signs of non-compliance or complications. This is particularly beneficial in rural or isolated areas where access to healthcare facilities may be limited. Remote diagnostics and treatment adherence monitoring could play a critical role in improving TB control, particularly in regions with high rates of the disease.

Treatment Innovations: New Drugs and Personalized Care

Historically, TB treatment has been lengthy, requiring patients to take a combination of antibiotics for several months. While effective, the traditional regimen is difficult for many patients to complete, particularly in low-resource settings. However, in recent years, several new drugs and treatment strategies have been developed to improve patient outcomes and reduce the duration of treatment.

Shorter and More Effective Regimens

One of the most promising advances in TB treatment is the development of shorter treatment regimens. In 2019, the World Health Organization (WHO) endorsed a new 9-12 month regimen for drug-sensitive TB, significantly reducing the treatment time compared to previous protocols. This shorter regimen has been shown to be as effective as the traditional six-month course, with fewer side effects, making it more accessible for patients in areas where healthcare infrastructure is limited.

For drug-resistant TB (DR-TB), new medications such as bedaquiline and delamanid have shown great promise. These drugs are part of a new class of TB treatments that target the bacteria in innovative ways, increasing the chances of successful treatment for patients who were previously untreatable. Clinical trials are ongoing to evaluate the efficacy of these medications in combination with other drugs to create more effective treatment regimens.

Personalized Medicine

The future of TB treatment may also lie in personalized medicine. By using genetic testing and molecular profiling, healthcare providers can determine the specific strain of TB a patient has and tailor treatment accordingly. This personalized approach could improve treatment outcomes, reduce the risk of drug resistance, and shorten the duration of therapy.

Research into the pharmacogenomics of TB treatment is still in its early stages, but it holds immense potential. By identifying genetic variations that affect how patients metabolize TB medications, personalized treatments could optimize drug dosages and minimize side effects. This would mark a significant step forward in ensuring that every patient receives the best possible treatment for their unique needs.

Preventing Tuberculosis: Vaccines and Public Health Strategies

Prevention is always better than cure, and in the case of tuberculosis, vaccines and public health measures remain the cornerstone of global control efforts. The development of a more effective TB vaccine and the implementation of comprehensive public health strategies are crucial to stopping the transmission of TB.

The Quest for a Better Vaccine

The Bacillus Calmette-Guérin (BCG) vaccine, developed in the early 20th century, remains the only licensed vaccine for TB. While BCG is effective in preventing severe forms of TB in children, its efficacy in adults, particularly against pulmonary TB, is limited. This gap in protection has driven a global effort to develop new and more effective vaccines.

Several promising candidates are currently in clinical trials, including the M72/AS01E vaccine and the VPM1002 vaccine. These vaccines have shown encouraging results in early-stage trials, offering the potential to prevent TB in adults and provide long-lasting protection. Researchers are also exploring novel approaches, such as DNA vaccines and vaccines that target specific strains of TB, which could provide broader immunity.

The development of a universal TB vaccine that offers protection across all age groups and against all forms of TB would be a game-changer in the fight against the disease. However, producing such a vaccine is a complex challenge, requiring ongoing research and substantial funding.

Public Health Strategies for TB Control

In addition to vaccines, public health strategies play a critical role in preventing the spread of TB. The WHO's End TB Strategy, launched in 2014, aims to reduce TB deaths by 95% and the incidence of TB by 90% by 2035. The strategy focuses on ensuring access to early diagnosis and treatment, promoting effective infection control measures, and improving the quality of life for TB patients.

National TB programs are working to integrate TB care with other health services, such as HIV and maternal health, to ensure that TB diagnosis and treatment are not isolated but part of a broader, more holistic approach to healthcare. The use of digital tools, including contact tracing apps and patient management software, can help public health workers identify and track cases more effectively, ensuring that all individuals who may have been exposed to TB are tested and treated promptly.

In high-burden countries, strategies to improve access to healthcare, reduce overcrowding, and promote better nutrition and hygiene are key to reducing TB transmission. Social protection programs that provide financial support to those affected by TB can help alleviate the economic burdens of the disease, enabling individuals to seek treatment and adhere to care regimens.

Overcoming the Challenges: Political Will and Global Cooperation

While innovations in TB diagnosis, treatment, and prevention offer hope, the continued success of TB control efforts depends on political will and global cooperation. TB is a global problem that requires a collective response from governments, international organizations, and civil society.

Sustained Funding and Commitment

The fight against TB has long been underfunded, with many countries struggling to allocate sufficient resources to control the disease. To end TB, global funding must increase significantly, particularly for countries with the highest TB burdens. Investment in research, healthcare infrastructure, and social services is essential to ensure that progress continues and that new tools and strategies can be effectively implemented.

The Global Fund to Fight AIDS, Tuberculosis and Malaria, the Stop TB Partnership, and other international organizations play a crucial role in mobilizing resources and providing technical assistance to countries in need. However, governments must also prioritize TB control within their national health agendas and ensure that TB is integrated into broader public health programs.

Strengthening International Collaboration

TB is a disease that transcends national borders, and its control requires collaboration between countries. International cooperation is essential to share knowledge, resources, and best practices, as well as to coordinate efforts to prevent the spread of drug-resistant strains.

The WHO's Global TB Programme, the Global Fund, and other entities provide a platform for countries to work together toward shared goals.

In addition, partnerships between governments, non-governmental organizations, the private sector, and the scientific community are vital to accelerating progress. By working together, stakeholders can overcome the challenges of TB control, ensuring that every individual, regardless of their economic status or geographic location, has access to the tools and treatment needed to prevent and cure TB.

Conclusion: A Path Toward a TB-Free World

The fight against tuberculosis is far from over, but with the advances in science, medicine, and technology, the prospect of a world free from TB is becoming increasingly realistic. Through continued innovation in diagnostics, treatment, and prevention, coupled with a commitment to addressing the social determinants of health, TB can be controlled, and ultimately eradicated. However, this will require sustained investment, political will, and global cooperation.

As we move forward, it is essential to remember that TB is not just a medical issue but a social and economic one as well. By addressing the underlying causes of TB, such as poverty, inadequate housing, and lack of access to healthcare, and by combating stigma and discrimination, we can ensure that all individuals have the opportunity to live free from the burden of tuberculosis.

The future of TB is one

Of hope, innovation, and global solidarity, and with the continued dedication of individuals, organizations, and governments worldwide, the end of the TB epidemic is within reach. The road ahead may be long, but with concerted effort and perseverance, a TB-free world is possible.

Printed in Great Britain
by Amazon